Alkaline Diet

Delicious Recipes That Are Suitable For People With GERD And LPR That Will Ease Your Heartburn And Make You Feel Better

(Build An Alkaline Body With Potassium And Sodium By Eating Potassium-rich Foods And Keeping Your Salt Intake To A Minimum)

I0089873

Dominique Pelletier

TABLE OF CONTENT

What Precisely Does One Consume When Following An Alkaline Diet?

Because there are so many crash diets out there, many people who are dieting choose to skip meals rather than stick to their regimen. Then, there are a lot of people who are trying to lose weight who have heard about the alkaline diet. However, what exactly is this diet? Fresh vegetables, fruit, nuts, and legumes are the primary components of this particular eating plan. It seems to be rather easy, doesn't it? On the other hand, if you are not aware of the scientific reasoning behind why this is effective, you could consider this to be simple logic. The book immediately dives into Alkaline-related topics.

An Overview of the Alkaline Diet's Past

1

This diet is founded on the presumption that our predecessors consumed a variety of foods that do not exist in our modern diet. Cheeseburgers and other forms of manufactured food were not available to hunter-gatherers. Their meals often consisted of both plants and animals, and this had nothing to do with the fact that their food was prepared. When compared to the nutrition of our predecessors, the modern diet has undergone enormous transformations.

After the invention of stone tools, grains were eventually included into the diets of our ancestors. Once equipment for sifting and rolling were developed, it became possible to get grains that had been refined.

As soon as domestic cattle became an integral part of their way of life, new foods such as milk and milk products like cheese were introduced into their meals.

The advancement of mining technologies and the expansion of accessible modes of transportation both contributed to a rise in the amount of salt that was consumed.

Because of technological advancements, more people are eating meat. Because of the advancements in technology that made it possible for cereals to be fed to cattle. Because of this, the cattle were able to swiftly gain weight.

At the beginning of the Industrial Revolution, there was a rise in the amount of sugar that was consumed.

According to the study that was conducted on this particular diet, practically all of the meals that are consumed, once digested, absorbed, and then metabolised, release either an alkaline or acid base into the blood. This occurs after the nutrients have been metabolised. Because fish, wheat, chicken, pork, cheese, shellfish, and milk as well as salt all create acid, it follows that the introduction of these sorts of foods and the huge growth in consumption of these types of foods meant that the Western diet had become more acid generating. In the end, there was a reduction in the consumption of vegetables and fruits, which contributed to the worsening of the effects of the diet high in acid generating foods.

Already, the blood has a very modest alkaline balance. The pH level should be between 7.35 and 7.45 on a scale from 0 to 14. The researchers on the alkaline diet indicate that the levels of alkalinity that are specified should be reflected in one's food. The proponents of this diet hold the idea that eating a diet that is rich in the sorts of foods that produce acid may throw off the pH balance of the body and can increase the loss of minerals such as magnesium, potassium, salt, and calcium. This is the theory that underlies this diet. Because of this imbalance, a person is more likely to get a variety of serious ailments.

Foods That Steal Your Energy And Make You Feel Tired

A healthy balance is essential to good health. This equilibrium is achieved when the body has a high concentration of alkaline minerals and a low level of acidic minerals. Because of this, it is essential to limit the quantity of acidic meals you take in while simultaneously increasing the proportion of alkaline foods in your diet.

You may change the internal equilibrium of your body by using the list of acidic meals that is provided below. Maintaining a healthy alkaline-acid balance is your objective. The upshot of this equilibrium will be improved health, increased vigour, and a general feeling of well-being.

Foods That Are Acidic

Drinking alcohol

Tea, coffee, and caffeine

Cocoa and chocolate both

Sweet honey

Szechuan Sauce

The perfect combination of vinegar and mustard.

Juice from fruit

Fruit that has been dried.

An excessive amount of fruit (how harmful this is also dependent on its sugar content).

There is beef, chicken, and pork.

Eggs

The shellfish

Cheese, milk, and every other dairy product

Various types of Mushrooms

Grains like wheat, oats, and rice are examples.

Excessive amounts of nuts and seeds, as well as sugar in all of its forms

foods that have been processed and packed

Ingredients and compounds that are synthetically produced.

The majority of items that have labels on them

Your life will be much improved if you cut down to a minimum on acidic meals or, more effectively, get rid of all of the acidic items on this list and replace them with an abundance of alkalizing foods. In any case, you should do this. You are going to be astounded by how easily your body may change into the fit and lively version of yourself that you have always envisioned becoming.

Always Prioritise The Consumption Of Vegetables.

The finest meals that nature has provided for human consumption are vegetables. Consuming a diet rich in vegetables may give you with a natural source of the nutrients that your body needs to perform at its best. Vegetables have quickly risen to the top of my list of must-eat items, and I believe they can do the same for you.

Vegetables are plentiful, easily accessible, and come in a broad variety of flavours and consistencies. There is a vast variety of flavours available in vegetables, and there are many methods to cook and enjoy these vegetables.

Because of their great nutritional value and low calorie content, they provide the body just what it needs to function properly. Consuming an excessive amount of calories and food that is low in nutritional value disrupts the normal rhythm of the body, leading to both weight gain and illness. Consuming nutrient-dense meals on a daily basis, such as vegetables, can help you reverse these conditions, allowing you to lose weight, feel healthier, and achieve a state of equilibrium.

Replace the foods that are on the list of acidic foods that you are going to start cutting out of your diet with the foods that are on the list below. If you want to see a significant improvement in your health, energy levels, and general well-being, try gradually switching from eating acidic meals to eating alkalizing foods.

Foods that are alkalizing

Produce of every sort that is organically grown

Fruit with a low sugar content

Nuts and seeds, especially those rich in water content (in measured quantities).

The grain quinoa

Barley grass and wheatgrass both

Kale

The spinach.

Herb parsley

The herb cilantro

The broccoli

Sprouts of lucerne.

Juice made from green vegetables and green smoothies (without any additional sugar)

Avocados

Beets ()

Carrots /

Cayenne pepper

It's a celery.

vegetables with dark green leaves, such as kale and collard greens

All varieties of organic lettuce.

The onion

Daikon radishes

Citrus fruits, lemons and limes

Artichokes Endives Endive Endive Artichokes

The asparagus

Sprouts of the Brussels

Cauliflower Baby potatoes
Cauliflower Baby potatoes

Coconut Grapefruit (Singular: coconut grapefruit)

Olive oil, as well as coconut oil

Visit the farmers' market in your neighbourhood. By purchasing goods produced locally, you not only help your community but also ensure that you have access to the freshest products possible.

When you go grocery shopping, you should acquire the majority of your food from the produce area, and you should always make an effort to buy organic versions of fruits and vegetables. Foods that have not been cultivated using organic methods may have been treated with harmful chemicals and pesticides. This indicates that you are taking in these poisons, which forces your body to exert more effort in order to expel them. Organic foods do not have any harmful chemicals or pesticides added to them. Although they may be more expensive, maintaining your health will save you the money that you otherwise would have to spend on medical expenses.

Cellulite is an unmistakable indication of an excessive amount of toxicity. They tend to manifest themselves most often on the buttocks, thighs, and belly. Cellulite may be treated with a wide variety of topical treatments, including lotions, creams, tablets, and even potions. The reality is that they do not. Put aside some of your cash. Invest it instead on nutrients that alkalize the body.

Your cellulite will disappear if you consume a diet that is mostly composed of green vegetables and if you make sure to eat some with each meal. Get enough of water in your system and stay away from meals and beverages that are acidic. In a short amount of time, your skin will get clearer, you will lose weight, and both your health and energy will improve. You will be surprised by how well rested and energised you feel, as well as how beautiful and young you appear, if you have patience and remember that the body and nature do not move quickly.

6. Dropping Pounds While Adhering to an Alkaline Diet

How to make the most of the alkaline diet to achieve your weight loss goals:

The alkaline diet is particularly effective at helping people lose weight, which is important since obesity is often associated with bodies that do not have a pH that is balanced. Lack of a balanced pH almost often indicates that the body is suffering from excessive acidity. The most effective treatment for balancing these acids would be to resort to an alkaline diet for rapid results. The alkaline diet does not include intense workouts, and it essentially only consists of monitoring what you eat.

Why put your faith in the alkaline diet as a way to get rid of excess fat?

The alkaline diet consists of natural foods and vegetables, and the following characteristics of these fruits and vegetables make them conducive to weight reduction on the alkaline diet.

• They include natural fats and sugars. • They contain natural vitamins, fibres, and minerals such as high amounts of iron, phosphorus, magnesium, and potassium. • They contain natural oils and sugars. • They contain natural vitamins, fibres, and minerals.

• They contain a significant amount of water.

• There is just a trace amount of sugar present in them.

• They are the manufacturers of acids such the amino acids and lycopene, which generate gastric fluids to dilute the effects of the acids.

• They contain a high amount of the antioxidant carotene.

• It is possible to consume them when they are still raw.

Consuming alkaline meals is associated with higher energy levels.

The meals listed below are widely recognised for their ability to provide energy; their names and the reasons why they produce high levels of energy are provided below.

The spinach.

Spinach, much like Popeye the Sailor, is well-known for its ability to boost one's energy levels due to the presence of several vitamins, minerals, and proteins that it contains.

Broccoli Broccoli is a fantastic source of energy since it contains a wide variety of nutrient-dense components, including zinc, manganese, and phosphorus, amongst others.

It's a celery.

In spite of its naturally sweet taste and high nutritional content, it has a long history of use as an aphrodisiac and has been shown to increase fertility.

Yeast-free potatoes

They have natural sugar in them, which will get the body's energy going in the morning.

Carrots Carrots are useful for creating eyesight energy because they include elements that are important in both the aqueous humour and the retina. Carrots also contain vitamin A, which is necessary for healthy vision.

Fruit bananas

They include minerals like calcium and potassium, in addition to the natural sugars, which contribute to the rapid synthesis of energy in the body.

Mandarin oranges

They are essentially enhanced with naturally occurring sugars and water, both of which play an important role in the generation of energy.

Beanzasrojos

These are very rich sources of fibre, vitamins, and other minerals, all of which contribute to the body's generation of natural sugars like sucrose and fructose, which, in turn, contribute to the body's production of energy.

Consuming alkaline meals may aid with weight reduction.

The following meals are beneficial for helping the body lose weight because they are all very rich in alkaline minerals, which provides them the capacity to maintain a well-balanced pH and also remove the excessive acids, cholesterol, and fats that are found inside the body. Note that eating fewer calories does not automatically result in a reduction in body weight.

Carrots Cabbage

Pebbles of Paprika

Various types of Mushrooms

The onion

The potato

Tomatoes (n.)

The aubergine

Kale

>Medicinal uses of collard greens

>The garlic

Bibb lettuce

Cucurbitapepo

>Olive Goat milk Olive Goat milk

Drinks with a high alkaline content for increased energy levels

Juice from apples

The apples are peeled and then pressed to extract the juice, which is high in vitamins and includes the mineral boron, which helps to build bones. The juice is generated by pressing the apples.

Juice made from grapefruits

Produced by pulverising or squeezing the grape fruit, this fruit is an excellent source of energy due to the presence of natural sugars and vitamin C in its composition. It is often used as a treatment for breast cancer, in addition to tiredness and sleeplessness.

Juice made from beetroots

The beetroot root that is used to make beetroot root juice is crushed, which results in the juice's red colour. Beetroot juice has a low percentage of naturally occurring sugar and is also a preventative strategy for high blood sugar.

The milk of almonds

Almond milk is produced from almond seeds and has a white appearance. It is a wonderful source of energy since it has a low amount of sugar and none of the lactose that is found in natural sugar. The prevention of cardiovascular disease and maintenance of bone health are two of the many medicinal advantages offered by this food.

Herbal infusions and teas

Herbal teas include ingredients in them that boost brain function, making it more productive while also promoting a sense of tranquilly. Introduction

I want to congratulate you for buying this book and I'm grateful that you did so.

The alkaline diet will be discussed in the next chapters, and you will get all of the knowledge you want to get started with the diet. Although it is referred regarded as a "diet," in reality, it is a change of lifestyle that you may keep up for the rest of your life. It is a manner of eating that promotes improved health, and it may help you maintain a healthy level of weight if it is done correctly.

This book will begin by providing you with all of the information you need to know on the diet. You will have a complete comprehension of what it is and what it is capable of doing. Research is also analysed so that you may have a better understanding of what the scientific community has to say.

The next chapter delves a little more into biological topics. You will have a deeper understanding of how the body responds to acidic and alkaline conditions after you take this course. This is the point in the process when you get to see how this diet may be useful for your health by knowing how it can have positive effects.

The third chapter discusses the kinds of meals that are healthy for you to consume. In addition to this, you have the opportunity to see the effects that food has on your body. This is the first step in getting ready for this diet that you have chosen.

In the fourth chapter, you will learn some useful advice that will assist you in maintaining your new diet. When you reach chapter five, you will be given information on pH testing, as well as instructions on how to conduct tests at home. This is significant because it tells you whether or not you are successfully sticking to your diet.

The conclusion of this book marks the beginning of your alkaline diet adventure. You will get the meal plan in its entirety, along with some delicious dishes for you to test out. The alkaline diet lifestyle may be started off on the right foot with this 14-day regimen.

There are a lot of books on the market that are related to this topic, so I want to thank you once again for picking this one. Please take advantage of the fact that every effort has been taken to ensure that it is packed with as much relevant information as is humanly feasible.

How To Maximise The Benefits Of An Alkaline Diet Through The Application Of Holistic Health Methods

When it comes to lowering acidity levels in the body, holistic practises like meditation and yoga play a significant role.

There are other things than diet that might help reduce acidity.

One of the most significant contributors to the production of acid inside the body is stress.

While the lives of the twenty-first century enjoy the advantages of technology, there has been a commensurate increase in the amounts of stress that people experience. Worry and anxiety are common outcomes of demanding work, precarious financial situations, and the responsibilities of raising a family. Recent studies have shown that there is a significant correlation between stress and acidity in the body.

The Connection Between Anxiety and Hyperacidity

Cortisol is a hormone that is secreted in response to stress. This hormone is what sets off the "fight or flight" response and pushes your body into overdrive. It has been shown that cortisol is also accountable for the quantity of bile produced by the liver. A high amount of cortisol induces an excessive flow of bile, which then gets 'dumped' in the small intestine when a person is stressed out. This additional bile is one of the primary contributors of acid reflux.

In actuality, the term "bile acid indigestion" has been shortened to its more common form, "acid indigestion."

(cholesterol is also present in the bile). Medication and acidity suppressants are only able to mask the symptoms of acidity; they do not treat the condition's underlying cause.

The lowering of acidity caused by eating an alkaline diet is the fundamental advantage of switching to an alkaline diet. You may increase the positive effects of an alkaline diet on your health by engaging in supporting practises like meditation and physical activity.

The relationship between Working Out and Stress

Although stress is an unavoidable component of life, prolonged exposure to it may have deleterious effects not just on the body but also on the mind. You will have low levels of energy, diminished well-being, and impaired mental attention if you are under stress for an extended period of time.

Activity of a light to moderate intensity results in increased energy levels, improved sleep, less anxiety, and decreased stress.

Almond Milk Flavoured with Strawberry Roses

This "strawberry almond milk with roe water" is "extremely easy," "completely delicious," and "packed with nutrients." This recipe is suitable for anyone following a paleo diet and is raw and vegan.

ITEM(S) REQUIRED:

1 cup of raw almonds that have been soaked in oak for 12 hours, 3 cups of filtered water, and 14 cup of pitted dates that have been chopped up (see "ee note" for a sugar-free option).

3 cups of fresh strawberries, 2 teaspoons of pure rosewater, and plenty more for tasting.

A smidgen of the Celtic ea alt
INTRUCTION

In order to "soak" the almond, place the nut in a bowl made of glass or ceramic and cover it with filtered water. A large glass jar may also be used. A teaspoon of Celtic tea salt and a splash of fresh lemon juice or apple cider vinegar should be added to the mixture. Allow the contents of the container to "soak at room temperature for 12 hours" while the container is covered with a breathable kitchen towel.

Drain and dispose of the soaking liquid; you will not need this for the milk-making process. In order to remove the anti-nutrient and enzyme inhibitor, the almonds need to be rinsed many times.

Place the almonds that have been rinsed and filtered water in your blender. Blend on high for 30 to 60 seconds, or until the almonds have been completely pulverised.

To train, place a nut milk bag or a knee-high piece of sheer nylon hoiery over the opening of a glass bowl, jar, or jug. This will prevent the dog from escaping. After pouring the milk into the bag, gently squeezing it while twisting it closed is the best way to get the liquid through the bag. Remove the almond pulp from the shell. (You can dehydrate this to use in a smoothie, or to make a scrub for your body, or you can make crutch out of it.)

Clean out the container of your blender, then add the strained milk, the strawberries, the date, the rosewater, and the salt. Blend until smooth. Mix vigorously for thirty to sixty seconds, until the mixture is silky smooth and creamy.

Put the milk in a container that can be sealed and put it in the refrigerator. Activated almond milk (milk made with "oaked almonds") may be stored in the refrigerator for up to three days if the temperature is kept very low.

Step 5: Gradually replace the majority of the items in your present diet with alkaline options.

It should not come as a surprise to the majority of people that replacing poor food choices with better ones is an excellent strategy for: Gradually adjusting to new conditions and progressing from being weak to being strong.

Choose healthier options for your meals instead of the less healthy ones.

Be patient and give your body time to gradually adapt and become healthier over the course of some period of time.

This is the most effective way to bring about whatever change you want in your life. Food is your fuel, and if you choose the appropriate meals, you may see rapid improvements in the state of your health. At this point, you ought to be aware of the many nutritious options available to you; the issue is, however, whether or not you will really implement them.

Taste is one of the most important factors in people's food preferences. Changes to your taste receptors are inevitable, however, if you are willing to put in the effort required to eventually make eating genuine excellent food a regular part of your life.

Do you remember being forced to eat different things when you were younger?

Now, however, such shifts may be brought about gradually, allowing for sufficient time to develop a genuine appreciation for the taste of nutritious meals. When you make the switch to organic foods, you could find that you can't ever go back to eating processed meals.

So begin right now. First things first: munchies, then meals.

Step 6: Maintain a food and beverage log on a regular basis, and utilise it to fine-tune your findings.

Keeping a journal of the things you eat and the things you do every day is important information. A food diary should also include the following: Keeping a record of your daily pH levels as well as everything that you put in your mouth.

Include details such as workout routines and meal plans that have proven successful in helping you reach your weight reduction objectives.

Keep notes so that you may go back to them later to help guide you in making additional decisions that seem to benefit both you and your body.

✓When people ask you how you managed to acquire such glowing health and wellbeing, use this answer as a model for others to follow.

You may keep a journal of your daily activities, weight, the foods you consume, and significant events that need noting for the purpose of gathering data in the future.

If you are keeping track of your health and you are feeling great right now, you will be able to relive that day in the future by doing the activities that you performed at that period of time. This information may also be utilised to make rapid improvements, since if you see a problem area, you can use your notebook to zero in on it and determine exactly what the issue is.

You may also share your diary with medical specialists so that they can more easily evaluate the effects of the things you've been doing to your body.

Do not miss writing a diary since doing so is required for accurate record keeping and is a very vital component of this process; thus, you should not skip it.

A Savoury Blend Of Vegetables With A Hint Of Spicy

Ingredients:

1 ½ teaspoons of cumin powder

2 cups of cooked bean, rinsed and drained

2 ½ cups vegetable stock

3 teaspoon of lime juice

4 tablespoon of chopped up cilantro

2 tablespoons of vegetable oil

1 chopped up large sized onion

1 Poblanochili, seeded and chopped

1 red bell pepper, seeded and chopped

3 cloves of garlic, minced

1 ½ teaspoons of chili powder

Instructions:

Bring a cooking pot up to a temperature that is just below medium. After pouring in your oil to heat it up, you should immediately add the onions to the pan so that they may be sautéed to perfection.

After everything else is finished, stir in the garlic, jalapenos, and Poblano and red bell peppers. Allow it to cook for approximately two to three minutes, or until all of the veggies have reached the desired degree of tenderness.

After that, put in the spices and mix everything together with a light hand. Along with the vegetable stock, include the beans into the dish.

Bring the whole mixture up to a boil, then continue to cook it for roughly 15 minutes at a temperature between medium-high and high. The lemon juice should then be stirred in, and some cilantro should be sprinkled on top as a garnish.

A helpful hint is that if you want to make the meal tastier, you could add some more ingredients immediately before you throw in the beans. These additional components may include cabbage, mushrooms, burdock, sweet potatoes, and so on. Because dairy, sugar, and animal items have the potential to reduce the amount of alkalinity produced by the recipe, it is imperative that none of these ingredients be used.

Water with an Alkaline pH

One more thing that is important to bring out is that many people feel that drinking alkaline water (which has a pH of 9.5 as opposed to the pH of pure water, which is 7.0) is healthier based on similar logic as the alkaline diet. Pure water has a pH of 7.0. In any case, it is not the case. The use of water that is too alkaline may be harmful to one's health and cause a disruption in one's nutritional balance.

If you drink alkaline water on a regular basis, it will reduce the amount of acid that is produced in your stomach and enhance the alkalinity of your stomach. Your capacity to digest food and absorb nutrients and minerals will decrease over time as a result of this condition. When there is less acidity in the stomach, it will make it easier for germs and parasites to enter the small intestine. This may be harmful to your health.

The conclusion is that drinking alkaline water is not the solution to achieving optimal health. Do not fall for any of the tricks used in marketing. Rather of doing that, you could put money into a reliable water filtering system for your house. Water that has been purified by filtration is still the healthiest option for your body.

Foods That Naturally Reduce Mucus Intake

Foods that help reduce mucus

putting it in its most basic form. It's safe to assume that most of us find mucus fluid to be repulsive. Surprisingly, it's really a quite clear result of our body's attempts to protect itself. Does that sound strange?

Take a look at this: just as it sheds tears and spits, the body also creates mucus fluid as a kind of self-protection. Mucous fluid, along with other natural liquids, contains a chemical that aids in the destruction of microorganisms that we come into contact with via the environment, the food we eat, or when our immune systems are under attack because they are vulnerable.

This is the reason why incompatible nutrition causes mucus, and this is also the reason why you make more mucus when you are sick. Therefore, even if it's not a very good idea, the liquid that the majority of people consider to be disgusting is really quite important to our survival.

The question at hand is whether or not we are consistently supplying mucus, which would indicate that the secure framework can dependably detect that it is being attacked. (This may also indicate that the tiny organisms in our gut are not as healthy as they should be since they protect us from pollution and unwanted microbes in situations when the body would not generate mucus anyhow.)

Therefore, in the event that we are producing a lot of mucus (postnasal dribble after eating, constantly running nose, cystic white skin break out, or persistent bodily fluid from the nose or eyes), we need to consider what we are consuming, what we are drinking, or what we are going through that is causing the response.

For certain people, the following foods are among the most allergenic:

Gluten, which is found in wheat and other grains, soy, dairy products, tree nuts, and eggs are all allergens.

For other individuals, the issue might be an illness of the immune system, a deficiency in basic zinc, or an inadequate amount of huge microscopic creatures. The first thing to do is figure out who is responsible for it, get rid of it, and then, if necessary, start an elimination diet.

Consuming an excessive amount of carbohydrates and refined sugar may similarly weaken excellent bacteria and, as a result, cause the body to produce mucus. Consequently, regardless of the nature of your circumstance, you should first attempt to make sense of it and then proceed to add this support underneath it.

Salad with Cucumbers and Basil

Perhaps one of the organic goods that gets the most cleansing out of its cucumbers. These are rich sources of water, potassium, and vitamin C, all of which contribute to the process of exfoliating the body.

In addition to enhancing immune health, vitamin C helps maintain healthy gut lining and reduces inflammation in the gastrointestinal tract, all of which are to the advantage of the immune system. Cucumbers have a fundamental nature that helps strengthen the gut lining.

Soup made with Broccoli and Coconut

Broccoli is an exceptional source of vitamin C and also includes catalysts that aid in the separation of toxins, so it's a double threat in terms of its ability to purge toxins from the body. Their fibre further takes care of beneficial microorganisms and assists in the removal of waste from the body, eliminating the need for detox tablets.

Millet with Fresh Vegetables of the Season

Carrots are an unpretentious root vegetable that are so common that it is easy to ignore their ability to nourish us on a fundamental level. Carrots have a high concentration of the antioxidant nutrient vitamin C, the essential electrolyte potassium, the bulk-forming carbohydrate fibre, and the nutrient A that is essential for maintaining a healthy immune system.

These root vegetables may be eaten raw or cooked, and they make exquisite dinner sides. This is preferable to eating processed wheat pastas and refined carbohydrates, which actually increase mucus production and weaken beneficial microbes.

Apple Pie in its Raw Form, Spiced with Goji Berries and Nutmeg

The vitamin C in apples and the kind of fibre known as gelatin give them their stellar reputation for helping to reduce the amount of fluid that the body retains. Apples' capabilities are only increased by their potassium level, and there are several ways in which one might enjoy eating an apple.

You may consume them, blend them, make juice with them, or heat them up. For a usually sweet treat, try concocting them with cinnamon and a few pears, or use fruit purée rather of sugar rather as butter and sugar in your next batch of cluster biscuits!

Cashew-Based Yoghurt Laced with Probiotics

Berries are yet another well-known organic food that may be used to exfoliate the body, especially the digestive system; however, this is not all they can do. Berries are an excellent source of vitamin C, potassium, and cancer-fighting antioxidants, in addition to being an excellent source of vitamin C.

These help clean the blood, and the fibre in them helps break down and remove toxins from the body, so reducing discomfort and pollution. Try making your next smoothie using berries like raspberries, blackberries, and blueberries rather of sweet sugars or sweet yoghurts. You may be surprised at how delicious it is!

They have a natural sweetness that lends the perfect flavour and will aid to support cell cleansing and immune system health in a natural way.

Overnight oats with Goji Berries and Chia Seeds

Due to the unique enzymatic properties that it has, ginger is able to expeditiously assist in the separation of toxins and physiological fluids.

It also has a neutralising effect on the body, which sends a message to the immune system that it is safe and that it does not need to produce a security component like mucus anyhow. This frees up the immune system to focus on fighting off the threat.

When possible, use fresh ginger, and if you want even more of the benefits of this remedy, try adding a tiny bit of turmeric. You may try them in a tea, a vegetable dish, or you could even squeeze them or blend them into a smoothie.

Salad with Kimchi and Kale

Greens are one of the most effective foods ever developed to aid in the recovery of the body. Greens include significant quantities of vitamins A, C, and B, as well as vitamin E and potassium, all of which work together to provide the body with support on every possible front.

Cook with greens in the evening, consume them throughout the day, or combine with them in the morning. All of these activities should take place during the day.

They naturally eliminate accumulated mucus and toxins, and their high fibre content will take care of beneficial microorganisms while their high chlorophyll content will support immune and blood health.

Water from a Spring

The use of a significant amount of spring water on a daily basis is essential to the success of the antacid diet. Seventy percent of an adult's body is made up of water. In order to operate correctly, the metabolic processes that make up the totality of the body need adequate amounts of water.Water helps the body eliminate waste, cushions the joints and organs, and facilitates the body's absorption of nutritional supplements.

The body's hydration levels as well as its electrolyte balance are best supported by drinking springwater since it naturally has alkaline and antacid properties. Springwater is also alkaline.

A Salad Of Chilled Green Beans With Fresh Lime

Ingredients:

1 tbsp. of Dijon mustard

2 garlic cloves, crushed

1 tbsp of lime juice

1 pound green beans, trimmed

¼ cup of extra virgin olive oil

Preparation:

Bring a saucepan of water to a boil, then stir in the green beans and one teaspoon of salt. Cook until the meat is soft. This should take around 10–15 minutes to complete. Drain and then rinse again.

In the meanwhile, mix the smashed garlic with some extra virgin olive oil, some Dijon mustard, and some lime juice. Serve the beans with the drizzle on top.

Delicious Sweet Potato Breakfast Bowl

Ingredients

½ tsp cinnamon to taste

If desired, almond puree, banana, peach and blueberries for garnish

300 g sweet potatoes

50 ml vegetable milk or water of choice

1 tbsp sweetener

Preparation:

To begin, cut the sweet potatoes in half lengthwise and then roast them in the oven for approximately thirty minutes, or until they are extremely tender. After the first 15 minutes of cooking time has completed, you should give them a single rotation.

After the sweet potatoes have had time to cool, you may peel them to remove the skin.

After that, place the sweet potatoes in a basin and use a fork to mash them until they are smooth.

At this point, more liquid may be added until the mixture reaches the appropriate consistency.

Cinnamon and any sweetener of your choosing may be used as a seasoning for this dish. Adjust the seasoning to your liking, and then top with almond paste, banana, peach, and blueberries, if that's what you'd like.

Ingredients

1 cup sautéed spinach (salt and pepper added, to taste)
½ a dozen cherry tomatoes

2 Portobello mushrooms
1 poached egg

Directions

Sprinkle a little bit of salt on the mushrooms and tomatoes after you have drizzled some olive oil over them.

Cook the tomatoes and mushrooms to perfection on the grill or in the oven until they are well done.

Add on a platter along with the egg, and then top with the spinach.

Have fun!

Smoothie Including Blackberries, Tofu, And Protein.

Ingredients:

- 8 ounces soft silken tofu
- 2 cups almond milk or more according to the consistency you desire
- 1 cup black berries
- 2 tablespoons honey or to taste
- 1 large banana, peeled, sliced

Method:

Put all of the ingredients into the blender, and run it until everything is completely smooth. If you want the smoothie to have a thinner consistency, you may make that happen by adding extra milk to the mixture.

Pour into large glasses, then top with crushed ice and serve immediately.

In What Ways Are These Foods Comparable To Drugs?

As I've said before, the compounds that are present in meals such as high-fructose corn syrup, casein, fats, and salts have chemical structures that ultimately make their way to our brains. As soon as they arrive, they search for extremely precise locations to relax in. Because these locations are constructed in the form of a puzzle, the chemicals that are looking for their "matching puzzle piece" in the brain are able to locate it and firmly attach themselves to it due to the fact that their structures perfectly complement one another. Exactly the same thing happens with medicines. When we take an opioid in the form of a narcotic, such as oxycodone, this opioid finds its way to the brain and has the same effect. It will search for the piece of the jigsaw that corresponds to itself and then closely bind to that component. The issue is that the chemicals that are found in food and those that are found in medications with a high potential for addiction are extremely similar; these will discover the same pieces of the jigsaw as each other. Because of this, they have the effect of making us feel exactly the same as one another.

They make us feel joyful, exuberant, and thrilled, and they give us the impression that we are having a wonderful time. This sensation is what compels individuals who are hooked to drugs like painkillers or cocaine to continue using them even though they know it would just lead to worse withdrawal symptoms. This is the root cause of the addiction that results from using these medicines. The pursuit of these lovely sentiments that arise from a very genuine chemical response in our brains is more important than a deliberate choice to continue.

Why do we feel so happy when this chemical reaction has taken place? This is due to the fact that these medications have a rewarding effect on both the brain and the body. When these chemicals, whether they be medications or dietary additives, locate their corresponding puzzle pieces inside the brain, this matching of parts prompts the brain to produce yet another molecule. These chemicals may be thought of as puzzle pieces. The subsequent release of this second hormone is what gives our brain the impression that it has been rewarded for its efforts. When we experience gratification, we have a sense of accomplishment, happiness, and excitement. Receiving the sensation that one has been rewarded is incredibly powerful and quite addicting for human beings. When our brain successfully matches together one of these puzzle pieces, we experience a satisfying sensation of achievement. Our brain is unable to distinguish between the effects of a medicine and those of an additive in food. Our brain is only aware of the fact that a chemical link has been made, at which point it produces the neurotransmitter associated with rewards. Because of this, it is quite hard to kick these addictions. People appear to have a general understanding that there is more to drug addiction than just a lack of willpower on the part of the individual, and that this additional factor is something that requires a great deal of effort to overcome. When it comes to food addiction, this concept is less well recognised as being synonymous with the same thing. When I describe this chemical process to you in this chapter, my intention is that it will help you understand why you have difficulties stopping yourself if you suffer from binge eating or why it is so difficult to say no when you feel like turning to food as a consolation. If you have binge eating disorder, you may find it difficult to stop yourself from eating.

Cane sugar

Now, let's take a closer look at sugar and the ways in which it influences both our bodies and our thoughts. Sugar is the most harmful of all of these food additives, and it should be avoided at all costs. This is due to the fact that avoiding it is really difficult! Sugar can be present in every single food that we consume, regardless of whether it was purchased from a restaurant or a shop. Because sugar may be found in so many different forms and is known by so many different names, it is often masked in the ingredient list on food packaging. A single food item may have seventy percent sugar in it, but the label may make it seem as if this is not the case. This is because the many forms of sugar have been broken out into their own categories so that we will believe that this is not the case. When it comes to staying away from sugar, you need to be very diligent and keep a close watch on the details.

We have previously spoken about one kind of sugar, which is High Fructose Corn Syrup (HFCS). This sort of sugar is inexpensive and simple to work with, and as a result, it is put to almost everything that is packed and that we may consume. This is because it provides a delicious flavour balance, even to dishes that are high in salt content.

The Use Of Sugar As A Drug

As was said before in this section of the book, the chemicals that are present in food have an effect on our brains that is very similar to the effect that extremely addictive narcotics have. Sugar itself operates in a certain manner, which is one of the reasons why it is so hard to resist. Sugar has an effect on a system that is referred to as the Limbic System. A set of structures in the brain known as the limbic system are responsible for our emotions and memories. These structures are located deep inside the brain. This involves the management of our emotions as well as the formation of our memories, both of which contribute to our capacity for learning. This indicates that the molecules that make up sugars might have an effect on our feelings when we consume food that is highly high in sugar. When something like this occurs, it triggers a range of feelings, including enjoyment and a sense of accomplishment. Then, since consuming certain meals causes us to experience such feelings, we create a memory of these experiences, and as a result, we learn that consuming particular foods causes us to feel in a favourable manner. Because of this, we can't help but come back for more.

Therefore, when we consume anything that has both sugars and casein, for example, there will be an effect on the limbic system as well as the reward system that is located in the brain. As a result, meals that provide us with both a sense of satisfaction and an outpouring of pleasant emotion are the ones that are the hardest for us to say no to, and the ones that we go for first when we are in need of solace in the form of food because we are certain that they will make us feel good. They do this each and every time because these chemical changes in the brain take place each and every time. Because it has become so ingrained in our habits, we may not even be aware of this anymore. It's possible that we don't recognise the good emotions that we experience after eating something that soothes us, but we are aware that we continue to want it for some unknown reason. If anything like this has ever occurred to you, you now understand the reason why it did. After being aware of these factors, pay attention to your desires and determine whether or not this might be the reason you experience them in the first place. You should also pay attention to the times of day when you have these desires. Have you recently heard some disheartening news? Was it a cloudy day when you were experiencing particularly negative emotions? Keep this knowledge handy since we will be using it again very soon. We will also be covering numerous techniques to overcome these obstacles later on in this book in order to stop the patterns of emotional eating and overeating.

21 Tricks To Get Your Ph Back In Balance

Since you now have an understanding of the fundamentals of the Alkaline Diet and also have an idea of what food kinds are the cornerstone of your diet, you are now prepared to tackle your diet head-on now that you know what the pillars of your diet are. Learning the 21 inner truths that are the keys to advancement on the Alkaline Diet is how you will be able to accomplish this goal. These exclusive insights will not only assist you in better acquiring the diet, but they will also reiterate the key notions that are necessary for entering your diet like Clark Kent and exiting it like Superman. It really isn't that much of a challenge.

The first key to restoring a normal balance in the body and enhancing overall health is to have an understanding of what pH is and how it functions. This is the foundation of a healthy body. Certain food kinds that we consume may either support the normal homeostasis that the body strives to maintain or disrupt it. This is because the human body strives to sustain a certain equilibrium.

Understanding what pH is and why it's important to one's health is necessary in order to make any headway when following the Alkaline Diet. This understanding is the key to success on the Alkaline Diet. Certainly, the vast majority of us would have learned about pH in school, but that was quite some time ago for a large number of you, and one of the goals of this book is to take what you know (and perhaps what you don't know) and assist you with diverting that data towards a healthy, more joyful way of life. Another objective of this book is to take what you know (and perhaps what you don't know) and help you with balancing your pH levels. Although it is not necessary to measure the pH of urine or other natural liquids in order to make success on this diet, you actually do need to have an important grasp of what is in different food kinds and why it is crucial. The good news is that we have already completed the great bulk of that work on your behalf by condensing all of that information into the two outlines that were presented in the previous chapter.

 The normal pH of the human body is somewhere in the range of 7.35 to 7.45, and this is our second little known secret. When the pH of the blood is below 7.35, it is said to be acidotic, and when the pH of the blood is above 7.45, it is said to be soluble or basic.

This is not a scientific book, and in order for the Alkaline Diet to be successful for you, you do not need to memorise any calculations. What is essential to understand, on the other hand, is that there is something that many people refer to as physiologic pH, and that is the regular pH that the body tries to keep up with in the blood and other extracellular liquids in order for it to take part in its generally expected substantial processes and accomplish homeostasis. Even though the pH might change depending on the kind of extracellular fluid, 7.4 is considered to be the normal range for the pH of blood. Remember that the body has to maintain this pH in order for proteins and other compounds in the blood to keep their regular form; this pH is also crucial for cells in the blood and lining the blood to participate in their usual metabolic and other activities. The body needs to maintain this pH in order for the body to function properly. Because maintaining this pH is essential to the continuation of life, the body must expend a significant amount of energy in order to do so.

3. Even ancient people understood the importance of consuming food sources that held a specific excess between the unique qualities of the food they were eating. This is the third and last hidden secret. The comparable concept is the foundation of the Alkaline Diet.

The underlying concepts behind the Alkaline Diet have been around for millennia, despite the fact that the modern version of this diet relies on science that was not definitely recognised until the beginning of the middle of the twentieth century. Even ancient people believed in something called "humours," which were essentially physical aspects of the blood and body that either contributed to illness or protected against it. Primarily, scientists and academics from the past were talking about pH as well as other synthetic features of the blood and the body, which we didn't start to understand until the twentieth century. These ancient brains were able to cure ailments with purely well-thought-out dietary regimens, despite the fact that we still struggle to adequately treat or even comprehend many of these conditions today.

People in the past were exceptionally wise in ways that we are unable to fathom, and they were able to have long, healthy lives by subsisting on naturally occurring soluble food sources such as olive oil, natural goods, vegetables, cereals, and grasses. This is in stark contrast to the situation in our times.

Secret No. 4: The modern Alkaline Diet is based on an unearthly ratio of 80% antacid detritus food kinds to 20% acidic food varieties.

The current Alkaline Diet, which we advocate for in this book, entails adhering to an eating routine that is made up of eighty percent of food sources that are considered basic debris and twenty percent of food sources that are considered corrosive debris. Although some people choose to follow a diet that consists of just but soluble detritus food choices, adhering to that restriction is not necessary when following this diet. As a consequence of this, in the event that you genuinely need to, you will want to consume some meat, fish, or eggs (along with other food sorts that fall inside the acidic range). The amazing thing about the soluble debris diet, and in contrast to what some people may believe, is that you are able to include a wide variety of tasty and energising food sources in this diet. This is something that you can do. This is not the diet your grandmother followed, which consisted of cod liver oil and prunes (both of which are acidic). Instead, this is a diet that allows you to easily include delicious meals on a regular basis. This is especially straightforward in the modern day, when food supplies and food products from all over the globe are more readily available than at any other time in history. Before we go on to the next mystery on the list, let's take a moment to talk about some of the delicious food selections that are available. We have compiled a list of 10 food sources that you may include into almost any supper in order to keep up with the alkalinity of the meal you are eating.

The grass of wheat. It is easy and uncomplicated to include a serving of wheatgrass into any meal, or even to take a shot at different intervals throughout the day. Wheatgrass may be easily bought at supermarkets and health food shops, and it only takes a few of efforts to a significant degree to gain the many medical benefits associated with this fantastic, easy soluble food. Wheatgrass is a superfood that contains a high concentration of chlorophyll.

Tofu . Tofu is not only a healthy and cost-effective dietary option, but it's also a versatile ingredient that can be used to a broad variety of dishes. Tofu, which is made from soybeans, is now more readily available than it has been at any point in recent history. You may bake it, eat it plain, or use it to create tofu burgers. Broiling is another option. Tofu is a supernaturally occurring food, and for certain individuals, it is also an essential component of the Alkaline Diet. The possibilities with tofu are virtually endless.

Nuts: almonds. The fact that almonds and other nuts are dry foods that are simple to transport and enjoy in nibble form is one of the many reasons why they are so popular. In addition, you do not need to nibble on them; rather, they may be an inherent component of a supper, comparable to a portion of mixed greens, a vegetable dish, and so on. The possibilities are endless. Not only that, but almond milk is also obtained from almonds, and it is a top option for those who are lactose intolerant or who want to keep things simple by eliminating creature milks (although, goat's milk is considered to be an antacid debris food). Almond milk can be found in grocery stores and health food stores. Almonds and almond milk are both components of a number of contemporary diets; hence, if you are actually committed to following one of these programmes, you should make excellent use of this component, which is almonds and almond milk.

Orange grapefruit. Grapefruit is not only delicious, but it also manages to be very accurate and robust in its presentation. Although it may seem as if those days are long gone, there is no need for them to remain so. People used to be interested in winding down on natural things like grapefruit, and although those days may appear to be in the distant past, they do not have to be. You will have a much easier time in meeting your day-to-day needs if you include grapefruit as one of the antacid trash food sources that you consume for the day, which should total 80 percent.

The seeds of sesame. A simple fundamental trash food that can be incorporated into any cuisine, sesame seeds are an excellent choice. They have a wonderful flavour, it is not difficult to get them, and they are not expensive. As part of your new Alkaline Diet routine, you may want to think about stocking your kitchen with some sesame seeds.

The fruit known as tomatoes. Tomatoes are a staple vegetable that the vast majority of you probably already know how to include into a variety of different dishes in your daily diet. It would not be much of a stretch to include them on a serving of salad greens or a tofu burger; alternatively, they might be consumed on their own as a snack.

The coconut. Coconuts are widely considered to be a superfood not just due to the fact that they are so nutritious, but also due to the fact that they are delicious and can be used in a wide variety of ways, allowing them to be included into a wide variety of meals and meal plans. Coconuts may be consumed in their natural state, but they can also be prepared into beverages such as coconut juice, coconut oil, coconut milk, and so on. We recommend making coconuts a regular part of your Alkaline Diet since they are a really miraculous food and because they help maintain a healthy pH level in the body.

Smoothie Made With Berries

Ingredients

1 cup of grapes, strawberries or frozen mixed berries

2 cups almond milk, unsweetened

2 cups fresh spinach

1 tablespoon chia

4 tablespoons almond butter, raw

1 banana, peeled and frozen

Directions

1. In a blender or food processor, puree the blanched spinach and almond milk until completely smooth.

2. Add the other ingredients, except the chia seeds, and mix until smooth.

3. When the mixture is smooth, add the chia seeds and continue to blend until they are fully incorporated.

4. Before serving, let the dish rest for a few minutes to let the flavours meld.

The Fatty Acids

A carboxylic corrosive with a long aliphatic tail (chain) that is either saturated or unsaturated is referred to as an unsaturated fat in the field of science, particularly in the field of organic chemistry.

The chain comprising the vast majority of naturally occurring unsaturated fats consists of a significant number of carbon molecules, ranging from 12 to 28.Triglycerides and phospholipids are the two main sources of fatty acids in the human diet.

Unsaturated fats are referred to be "free" fats when they do not have any other particles to which they are attached. Because of the high levels of ATP that are produced during the metabolic process of unsaturated fats, these fats are essential sources of fuel for the body.

For this purpose, a wide variety of cell types are able to make use of either glucose or unsaturated lipids. More specifically, oily acids are preferred by the heart and the skeletal muscle. In contradiction of long-held beliefs, it has been shown that brain cells, at least in some rats, may use unsaturated fats in addition to glucose and ketone bodies as a source of fuel. This is in addition to the fact that glucose is a known fuel source for brain cells.

Fatty acids may be divided into two primary categories: saturated and unsaturated.

Saturated fatty acids are characterised by the presence of carbon-carbon double bonds.

fatty acids that are not saturated and do not include double bonds.

Unsaturated fatty acids Unsaturated fats are distinguished from saturated fats by the presence of one or more double bonds between their carbon atoms. (Collections of carbon particles that are held together by twofold bonds may be soaked by including hydrogen iotas in the process, which results in the transformation of the twofold bonds into single bonds. As a consequence of this, the two-fold securities are referred to as unsaturated.)

It is possible for a cis or trans configuration to take place between the two carbon molecules in the chain that are bound by either side of the two-fold bond.

Cis

In a cis configuration, the two hydrogen iotas that are next to the twofold bond are located on the same side of the chain as the twofold bond.

Due to the presence of the cis isomer, the chain will twist, which will limit the conformational flexibility of the unsaturated fat. The inflexible nature of the double bond fixes the conformation of the molecule, making it more compliant.

The chain's flexibility decreases proportionately with the number of double bonds it has in its cis configuration. When a chain has a large number of cis bonds, the chain will turn out to be very twisted in the majority of its possible configurations.

For example, oleic corrosive has a "crimp" in it because it only has one twofold bond, but linoleic corrosive has a more pronounced curve since it has two twofold bonds. Both of these corrosives are oleic acids. A snared structure is supported by an alpha-linolenic corrosive molecule, which has three twofold bonds.

The effect of this is that, in constrained situations, such as when unsaturated fats are a part of a phospholipid in a lipid bilayer, or triglycerides in lipid beads, cis securities constrain the capacity of unsaturated fats to be firmly stuffed, and as a result, they can influence the temperature at which the layer or the fat softens.

Because of the increased intricacy of a trans arrangement, it is likely that the two hydrogen molecules that are located adjacent will be found on opposite ends of the chain. As a result, they do not cause the chain to twist very much, and their form is comparable to that of unsaturated fats that have been straight soaked.

In the majority of naturally occurring unsaturated fats, every double bond has three more carbon molecules after it, totaling some number "n," and all of these bonds are cis bonds. The vast majority of unsaturated fats in the trans configuration (trans fats) do not occur naturally and are instead the result of preparation by humans (for example, hydrogenation).

Saturated fatty acids: Saturated fats do not contain any double bonds. Because double bonds reduce the number of hydrogens that may bind to each carbon, this process results in unsaturated fats that are saturated with hydrogen. Because saturated unsaturated fats only contain a single bond, every carbon atom within the chain has two hydrogen molecules (with the exception of the omega carbon at the very end, which has three hydrogens).

Essential lipids that are unsaturated

The term "key unsaturated fats" refers to those types of unsaturated fatty acids that are essential for human health but cannot be synthesised in sufficient quantities from other types of substrates. As a result, these fats must be obtained from the diet.

There are two different configurations of essential unsaturated fats: one has a double layer of protection consisting of three carbon particles that have been eliminated from the methyl end, and the other has a double layer of protection consisting of six carbon molecules that have been eliminated from the methyl end. As shown when seen from the carboxylic corrosive perspective, it is not possible for people to form double bonds in unsaturated fats with carbon atoms beyond the 9th and 10th positions.

Linoleic acid, also known as LA, and alpha-linolenic acid, sometimes known as ALA, are two of the most important unsaturated fats. In most cases, they are spread by the oils of plants. The potential of the human body to convert ALA into the longer chain n-3 unsaturated fats eicosapentaenoic corrosive (EPA) and docosahexaenoic corrosive (DHA), both of which may also be obtained from fish, is somewhat limited.

Components of fats that are unsaturated in nature

Components of fats that are unsaturated in nature Fatty acids serve the body in four very important roles, which are as follows:

In the manner of constructing squares. Unsaturated fats are the basic components of phospholipids and glycolipids, which are the components that make up the layers of a cell.

In the interest of concentrating on particles. There is a connection between unsaturated fats and a variety of proteins. Along these lines, proteins are co-ordinated to fit into the appropriate location in films.

As particles used in fuel.Triacylglycerols, which are esters of glycerol and unsaturated fats, are the form in which unsaturated fats are stored. Triacylglycerols are also sometimes referred to as triglycerides or unsaturated fats.

Atomic messengers, also known as couriers. The consequences of the function of unsaturated fats as hormones and as intracellular errand person particles, also known as dispatchers.

Alkaline Baked Bean Salad Breakfast Casserole

Ingredients

2 handfulsofspinach

2 clovesofgarlic

1 avocado

½ lemon

Olive oil

1 dessert spoonof coconut oil

Himalayansalt&black pepper

1 canof haricot beans (pref. organic)

4 springonions

6 cherrytomatoes

1 handful of basil

Instructions

Prepare the spring onions by chopping them roughly, cherry tomatoes by cutting them in half, and garlic by chopping them very finely. Now, in a frying pan that is large enough, put a little amount of water to a boil (maybe fifty millilitres or less), and'steam fry' the garlic for one minute. Now, stir in the haricot beans, cherry tomatoes, and spring onion, and continue to cook until everything is tender.

After that, put in the basil and the spinach and cook it until it wilts. After that, season it with the Himalayan salt and the black pepper, and then put in the coconut oil and stir it.

While this is cooking, make a side salad and cut the avocado in half, and then you'll be all set.

The bean salsa mixture should be served with a salad and the avocado half, with lemon juice and olive oil drizzled all over the top.

A Salad Made With Avocado And Sprouts

2   tbsp.   fresh   lime   juice
4 tbsp. cold pressed extra virgin olive oil
Pepper   and   sea   salt
Some fresh basil

2   normal   sized   avocados
8oz.   tomatoes
5-6oz.   alfalfa   sprouts
1   clove   of   garlic

To prepare avocados, peel and cut them. Lime juice should be sprinkled on top. Before adding the tomatoes and lucerne sprouts to a bowl, chop the tomatoes and clean the sprouts. In a low-volume bowl, combine the olive oil, lime juice, and garlic that has been chopped very finely. Mix together the salt, pepper, and basil after adding them to the mixture. Avocados should be added to the sprouts before the dressing is poured on top. Combine thoroughly.

Myths Regarding The Alkaline Diet

The alkaline diet is sometimes referred to as the acid-alkaline diet and the alkaline ah diet. After being metabolised, the meals you consume are said to leave a "ah" residue behind in your body. This is the central tenet of the theory. The ah may either be acidic or basic in nature.

Certain meals, according to proponents of the diet, may change the acidity or alkalinity of physiological fluids such as urine and blood. These fluids include blood and urine. If you consume foods that contain acdc ash, they will turn your body into acdc. Consuming meals that contain alkaline ah will cause the body to become more alkaline.

On the other hand, alkaline ash is thought to be protective against diseases like cancer, osteoporosis, and muscle wasting, while acid ash is thought to make you more susceptible to these diseases. It is advised that you use convenient pH test strips to monitor the acidity level of your urine in order to ensure that you maintain an alkaline balance.

Diet claims that sound like this may be rather compelling to those who do not have a comprehensive understanding of human physiology and are not nutrition experts. But isn't that statement really accurate? In what follows, a common misconception about the alkaline diet will be busted, and some confusion will be resolved.

But first, it is essential to have a comprehension of the significance of the pH value. To put it another way, the pH value of anything is a measurement of how acidic or alkaline it is. The pH value may be anything between 0 and 14.

• 0-7 are considered acidic; 7 are considered neutral; 7-14 are considered alkaline

 For instance, the "tomach" may be loaded with extremely acidic hydrochloric acid, which may have a pH value ranging from 2.2 to 3.5. The acidity assists in the killing of germs and the digestion of meals.

On the other hand, the pH of human blood ranges anywhere from 7.35 to 7.45, and it is almost usually somewhat alkaline. In a normal state, the body uses a number of efficient processes, which will be discussed in more detail later, to maintain a blood pH that is within this range. The risk of falling out of it is quite high and may even be fatal.

The Impact of Different Foods on the Blood and Urine pH

When foods are burned, they produce either an acid or an alkali ash. Phosphate and sulphur are both found in ash from volcanic eruptions. Calcium, magnesium, and potassium are the elements that are found in alkaline.

There are food categories that are categorised as either acidic, neutral, or alkaline.

Foods that are acidic include meat, fish, dairy products, eggs, grains, and alcohol.

Sugars, carbohydrates, and fats are all considered neutral.

Fruits, vegetables, nuts, and legumes are all good sources of alkalinity.

pH of Urine

The pH of your urine may be altered by the foods you consume. If you have a green smoothie for breakfast, your urine will have a higher alkaline content a few hours later than it would if you had bacon and eggs.

The urine pH may be very easily monitored for someone who is following an alkaline diet, and the results may even bring instant gratification. Unfortunately, the pH of urine is not a reliable sign of the pH level of the body as a whole, nor is it a reliable predictor of one's overall state of health.

The Most Effective Alkaline Diet

You are able to lower the acid levels in your body. If you suffer from ailments such as cancer, arthritis, heart disease, stroke, or any number of other illnesses, your body is acidic. Acidosis is a condition that occurs when there is an excess of acid in the body, whether it be in the blood or in the tissues of the body. The pH level is the most important element in determining your overall health and the risk of developing disorders.

When cancer patients are analysed, it is discovered that their cells have very low oxygen levels and high pH acidity, both of which favour the growth of malignant cells. Cancer of the stomach, cancer of the colon, cancer of the liver, cancer of the oesophagus, cancer of the pancreas, and other sorts of malignancies and disorders might result from this.

Which foods are considered to be alkalizing?

The majority of an alkaline diet consists of fresh fruits and vegetables, certain low-calorie whole grains, nuts, seeds, oils, and a wide variety of other foods, all of which we have included for your convenience so that you may more easily take them on a regular basis.

As the old saying goes, "health is wealth." You have a responsibility to look after your own health as well as that of your loved ones. The treatment of a sickness may be taxing not just physically but also psychologically and financially. It is even capable of causing tension and despair, in addition to having an impact on interpersonal interactions.

In order to have happy and fruitful lives, everyone of us must take responsibility for our own lives as well as the lives of others we care about. Consuming the most alkaline diet possible is the primary means by which we may accomplish this goal.

The optimum alkaline diet strikes a balance between meals that are acidifying and those that are alkalizing, with the ratio being 20:80. Any surplus acids are neutralised and flushed out of the body by the body's organs, such as the liver and the kidneys. However, there is a limit to how much acid even a healthy body is able to neutralise and properly remove via the body's systems. This limit applies even to healthy bodies.

An excessive amount of acidity places a load on the body's systems, which must work harder to detoxify the acid. The human body is designed in such a manner that it is naturally capable of regulating its own acid-alkaline balance provided that the following conditions are met:

You eat an alkaline diet that is well-balanced and healthy.

The organs carry out their functions well.

It is important to prevent having an excess of acid in the body.

This is one of the natural strategies to keep up your fitness and maintain your vitality. Regrettably, the majority of people eat foods that contribute to an acidic environment in the body as their primary source of nutrition. These foods that produce acid put a burden on the body's mechanism for detoxification, which results in an accumulation of the acid in the body.

It is impossible for the body's processes to keep up with the labour required to eliminate excess acids from the body. It is essential for you to consume an alkalizing diet, since this will neutralise the acidity in the body and relieve stress on organs such as the kidneys and the liver.

Is It Essential To Have An Alkaline Water Ioniser?

In the most recent few months, a substantial quantity of information on an alkaline water ioniser that is suitable for use in the house has been made available.

It is thought that an alkaline water ioniser is able to ionise water, which delivers several health advantages to the drinker, including a delay in the ageing process throughout the human body. However, there is not a great lot of scientific evidence to support this theory.

This is a natural medication that is used in many different branches of natural medicine to not only slow down the ageing process but also help a person feel better after they have been afflicted with a sickness.

An alkaline water ioniser designed for use in the house is available for purchase if you are interested in acquiring a gadget of this kind. Without having to make a trip to the neighbourhood health food shop, these gadgets guarantee that you will always have access to the highest quality ionised water. Ionised water is very pricey to acquire on its own, not to mention the fact that you are going to discover that purchasing an industrial-sized device, which is a massive device that sits on top of a countertop, is going to be something that you do not want to do if you do not want to spend the thousands of dollars that the equipment often costs.

The good news is that these home-based machines can ionise one cup of water at a time, which means that you may reap the potential health advantages of the water without having to shell out as much cash for a more expensive machine.

Over the course of time, you will see that you have saved a significant amount of money in comparison to what you would have spent on buying individual water bottles or just going out and purchasing the bigger equipment. If you want to stay up-to-date on the most recent developments in the world of health goods, a water ioniser can be just what you need.

The formation of naturally occurring alkaline ionised water is the result of a filtering process that begins with the evaporating effects of the sun and then returns to the purifying effects of the earth via the action of rocks, sand, sediment, and the earth's magnetic fields on the numerous minerals that are present in streams, lakes, and subterranean wells. This process may take millions of years.

This produces what is known as "ph balanced water," which is water that is ideal for healthy consumption. That is, until we humans find a way to screw everything up.

As a result of the industrialization of the globe and humankind's never-ending need to improve their standard of life, we are unable to locate any source of totally uncontaminated and pure alkaline ionised water anywhere in the world at this time.

Because the earth has such an incredible system for transporting its naturally existing alkaline minerals to all locations on the surface of the planet's oceans, it also transports all of the man-made chemicals that we produce to all locations in the same way.

Today, these hazardous and lethal substances have been discovered even in the most inaccessible and purportedly "untouchable" regions, such as the deepest jungles of the Amazon and the subterranean waters of the Sahara desert. They have even been discovered locked away in the top layers of the polar regions of Antarctica and the Arctic.

Imagine the contaminants that are present in the water of developing nations who have insufficient or nonexistent water treatment facilities. Aren't you happy that most developed nations, including the ones in which we live, have municipal water filtration systems that ensure that 'our' water is clean? Don't be too sure!

According to the findings of a number of studies, the tap water in our kitchens and bathrooms contains a variety of man-made compounds, many of which are very acidic. Some of it comes from the municipal systems that were specifically designed to maintain the 'cleanliness' of the water that we use for drinking and bathing. They are required to be included in the system due to the requirement of preventing the water from getting contaminated with illness when it is transported through the pipe system to our houses and then eventually comes out of our taps.

However, as we would prefer not to consume these ostensibly "beneficial" substances, we install filters on our sinks and in our refrigerators in an effort to get water that is free of impurities and may be considered "pure."

In the end, however, there are literally hundreds of chemicals that find their way into the water we use for drinking and bathing at some point, and there is no filtering system or process that has been created by man that would totally rid us of 'all' toxins in our water. Simply put, we make the most efficient use of the resources at our disposal.

When we return to the way nature intended things to be, we discover that the original source of life-giving water was really made up of many minute quantities of beneficial alkaline minerals; minerals that our bodies need.

The interaction of these minerals with the earth's natural magnetic fields resulted in the water having a natural ionising effect, which caused the water have a nature that was just slightly more alkaline. That is, at a level that is slightly higher than neutral on the pH scale, which is 7. This was the manner that mother nature provided us with ionised and alkaline water. Water that has a ph that is just right.

A matter of private opinion

I do not have a degree in medicine or any other professional field. I am just a lady who has struggled with a variety of health issues in the past and who has only very lately been aware of the concept of alkaline ionised water having potential benefits for one's health. It made perfect sense to me at that very moment since, many years before, I had really seen with my own eyes living blood molecules from my own body moving about and colliding with each other on a computer screen. What I saw really captivated my attention. The fact that my blood was very acidic, as opposed to the slightly alkaline level that is considered to be healthy, was another thing that disturbed me about the results.

The physician said that in a perfect world, all of my blood molecules would be isolated from one another and would easily bounce off of one another. The majority of mine were in a 'chained' position. We are entangled with one another like links in a chain, making it difficult for us to move around.

In addition to this, I saw in my blood what seemed to be crystals with points and sharp edges, and I was informed that these are the consequence of years of having high quantities of acidic substances in my blood. In addition to that, I saw what seemed to be a bizarre underwater starfish-like creature with five or six lengthy tentacles swimming about. It was a moving object. I was informed that this particular sort of parasite was rather frequent in patients who had blood that was extremely acidic.

An acidic environment is "ideal" for the growth of parasites and many other illnesses. They either cannot live in an alkaline environment or, if they can, they do not like living there. Because of this, nature has endowed us with naturally occurring alkaline ionised water that has a pH that ranges from slightly alkaline to slightly acidic.

The highly processed foods we consume, the water and soft drinks that include added chemicals, and the filthy air that we breathe on a daily basis are all doing our bodies no favours in the modern day.

Blood that permits all sorts of nasty things to 'thrive' and flourish while we go about our busy lives entirely ignorant of what's occurring in our bodies over the years is present in almost every individual in western civilization and in many other cultures in today's world by the time they reach adulthood. This is the case even for a large number of people living in other cultures.

And yet, we continue to be mystified as to why so many individuals in this day and age succumb to illnesses such as cancer and others. Cancer is one of those "nastiest" diseases that does not thrive in an alkaline atmosphere.

The most important information that you will find on this website is going to be about alkaline ionised water since it is founded on the concept that this kind of water may play a vital part in the efforts that we make to improve our health.

This website is going to focus on water, specifically alkaline ionised water, even if there are obviously many other methods to live a healthy life and "alkalize" our bodies. However, the primary focus will be on water.

I will make an effort to provide information in an order that makes sense, based on what I have discovered both from personal experience and via study. In this day and age, with so much pollution, I find it to be a really intriguing issue to discuss.

The following are some of the benefits of being alkaline and hydrated:

2) One of the fluid systems that is continually working to maintain a pH of 7.4 (slightly alkaline) is the circulatory system, which includes blood. If your body's pH is slightly alkaline, this implies that your blood cells and tissues are well oxygenated and that they are in the optimal position to neutralise and detoxify the waste products and toxins produced by your metabolism. As a result, you will be in a state in which you are:

vivacious and healthy physical form

A stronger immune system

High intensity of energy

Clarity of thought and strength of performance

bright and radiantly healthy looking skin

attitude of mind that is optimistic

The maintenance of a healthy pH balance is one of the most essential steps in developing a robust immune system and warding off disease in the early stages of infection. For instance, patents related to cancer are always toxic (there are no exceptions) and most of the time eating the incorrect food and experiencing emotional distress as well as other issues associated to stress.

The surroundings, the body fluids, and the body's humours are all referred to as the terrain. These make up 80% of the body and need a pH value between 7.2 and 7.6 in order for the proteins to assume the form of life-supporting bacteria and be used by the body. Because of disruptions in the flow of Meridian energy throughout the body, the pH value might be different in different locations. When the pH value changes, the protists transform into bacteria that are able to survive in an environment with a low pH and high activity.

Both metabolism and energy may serve interchangeably as the first or second source of environmental problems. The environment has two causes. They are able to change their life form, which is known as pleomorphism. Prota cannot be destroyed. Energy that cannot be destroyed equals a change in the flow of merdaan.

For instance, cholera germs need a pH of 6 (this figure is used for the sake of demonstrating the point).

If cholera germs get into the body, the body's 7.2 pH will cause the bacteria to mutate into a form that can survive at that level, preventing an epidemic of cholera. If the body's pH level is six, the cholera bacteria will flourish, and other bacteria in the body will convert into cholera bacteria as well. Because of this, some people are able to understand it while others are unable. To explain the connection between Metabolism and Meridian Energy, both of which are responsible for the Terrain, would need a presentation lasting more than one hundred hours....

Nothing can be kept a secret. 'Merck et al tets' every new antibiotic against the pleomorphic effect, so that they know into what kind of bacteria the cholera will change (another harmful one since it lives in the same pH 6 environment). They are aware that the only treatment is to lower the pH of the planet to 7.2, but this can only be accomplished via the body's metabolism, which requires healthy food as well as an uninterrupted supply of energy.

Energy That Is Pulsating Reoance Therapy (also known as PERTH)

Building up one's energy reserves and maintaining a healthy organ balance (PERTH)

Detoxification of the body in its whole, achieved by natural means and repeated use of

Treatment and prevention of over 200 different disease conditions are offered here.

Enhanced activity of the cell's metabolism

Bringing the blood pressure back to normal

What Are Some Natural Ways That You May Lose Weight?

Foods that have a high concentration of acid are often exceedingly harmful and frequently lead to obesity. Consuming meals that promote acid production has an effect on your body's ability to burn fat, as well as on the frequency with which you experience feelings of hunger. On the other hand, foods that promote an alkaline environment are thought to have an anti-inflammatory effect. This enables you to consume the appropriate number of calories while yet maintaining a sense of fullness after consuming them. Getting your weight under control and keeping it there are both aided by all of these factors.

The anti-aging effects of an alkaline diet, such as your skin seeming more young and supple, are just one of the many health advantages of a balanced alkaline diet. Additionally, it raises your levels of energy and mental alertness, while at the same time ensuring healthy digestion and improving the quality of your sleep at night.

To begin, it is essential to have a solid understanding of the manner in which acidic-forming meals have a detrimental effect on our bodies, which is mostly via the red blood cells. Red blood cells contain a mechanism that keeps them apart from one another and prevents them from clumping together. This is essentially a negative charge that keeps them apart from one another and serves as a barrier between them. Because it strips the red blood cells of their negative charge, an increase in blood acidity may cause this process to become dysfunctional. Because of this, the red blood cells in your body will begin to clump together, which will reduce the amount of oxygen that is able to reach your cells. Therefore, increased acidity in your blood may contribute to the deterioration and eventual death of red blood cells in your body.

Now, for a look at the advantages of eating an alkaline diet:

Fights Against Exhaustion

When there is an excess of acidity in your system, the availability of oxygen is reduced, which in turn hinders the capacity of your cells to repair damage and acquire nutrients. If your body is deprived of the nutrition it needs to produce energy, you will undoubtedly experience feelings of weakness. If you have been feeling sleepy and bewildered during the day despite getting the recommended amount of sleep, then it is possible that you need to examine the acidity levels in your body.

Increases one's resistance to illness

Your body's capacity to ward against infections caused by bacteria and viruses is diminished when the pH levels are out of whack. As a result of their being a deficiency of oxygen in the system (which is caused by acidity, as was just discussed), there is an increased likelihood of viruses and bacteria flourishing in the circulation. It is vital to alkalize in order to reduce or eliminate the risk of illnesses occurring.

Builds up your bone density.

Calcium is used up at a greater rate as individuals become older, particularly if they consume a diet that is high in acid-based foods. When we consume meals that are high in acidity, our bodies have to work to neutralise the acid by releasing calcium, magnesium, and phosphorus into the bloodstream. The vast majority of the time, the stocks of these minerals are withdrawn from the bones, which may be a significant issue in the long term. However, there is no need for your body to take these minerals from your bones if you follow an alkaline diet since you are not consuming fewer items that generate acids and hence your body will not have to. In addition, the many alkaline foods that are abundant in these minerals help you take in a greater quantity of these minerals via your diet.

A leaner and healthier physique in addition to weight reduction

The alkaline diet serves as the foundation for a diet that is generally rather healthy. To begin, the plan calls for you to cut down or eliminate alcohol, red meat, sweets, trans fats, and processed foods, all of which will unquestionably facilitate your weight reduction and provide you with a variety of other additional health advantages. Additionally, the diet encourages you to consume a greater quantity of fresh and nutritious meals, such as vegetables, fruits, and water, all of which improve your overall health and raise the likelihood that you will succeed in shedding extra pounds.

Acquiring Knowledge about pH

Now that you have a solid understanding of the fundamental principle of an alkaline diet, allow me to elaborate on the idea of "pH" levels.

It is really essential to have a solid comprehension of pH levels in order to better realise how the alkaline diet operates.

Therefore, in a broad sense, pH is a component of our blood that is referred to as the "Potential of Hydrogen."

It is possible to ascertain if a liquid is alkaline, acidic, or neutral by measuring the pH level of the liquid and comparing it to the appropriate scale.

When it comes to people, the acidity or alkalinity of bodily fluids and tissue is often something that is measured.

On a scale ranging from 0 to 14, the measurement is taken (see to the image to the right for reference). Reading the scale according to this common convention yields the following results:

When the pH value of a solution drops, the acidity of the solution increases.

The higher the number, the more alkaline the solution is. Increasing the value.

On the scale, 7 is the point that is regarded to be the neutral point.

The pH level of our bodies remains relatively stable around 7.4, which is the point at which it is believed that the body's mechanisms operate at their highest degree of effectiveness.

Researchers have established, however, that a moderate rise in the alkalinity level of pH tends to greatly enhance the general health state of the body. This is the case despite the fact that the rise is very minor.

However, the pH level of the body changes from one place to the next, which is something that has to be taken into consideration. For instance, many people believe that the stomach has a naturally acidic environment, making it the most acidic area of the body.

The human body, along with the bodies of a great number of other creatures, begins to respond unfavourably if the pH level that is naturally present in the environment is even slightly changed.

One notable example would be the recent rise in the disposition of carbon dioxide, which led to a significant minor fall in the pH of the ocean, bringing it down to 8.1 from 8.2 where it had been before. If there is even a 0.1 fluctuation in pH, then many different aquatic species and forms of life have already begun to suffer.

This pH level is not only vital for the development of plants, but it also makes up a component of the minerals that are found in the food we eat.

However, every biological organism has several mechanisms that may protect the body against these kinds of alterations. In the case of humans, several different minerals work together as a "buffer" to keep the pH level of our bodies at a healthy level, even if they grow more acidic.

The Emphasis Is On The Alkaline Diet.

A diet that is considered to be alkaline is one that helps keep the pH balance in the body at a level that is more alkaline rather than more acidic. As a result, you not only get healthier but also lose weight, which in turn reduces your likelihood of developing a variety of ailments. When nutritionists began publicly praising the efficacy of this diet and describing the ways in which adhering to the diet plan and making it a part of one's daily routine might help one live a longer and more fulfilling life, the diet acquired a great deal of popularity.

Understanding an alkaline diet may be quite difficult since, at first look, this diet seems to be highly intricate. This can lead to a lot of misunderstanding. In principle, eating an alkaline diet should help you reduce the acidic levels in your body.

There is a great variety of meals that may help lower the acid levels in your body. Because people are so used to making these acidic meals a regular part of their diet, they are unaware of the effects that it is having on their body. If you have been following a normal diet plan, you may have seen that you have shed a few pounds, which may give you the impression that you have found the answer to all of your weight loss problems.

Despite this, there is no assurance that you are making progress towards a healthy lifestyle. If you want to maintain your health, you need to reduce the likelihood that illnesses may develop in your body and ensure that your important organs continue to operate well. This is what an alkaline diet accomplishes for you, and it is for this reason that once individuals learn how successful the diet plan is, they begin shifting towards an alkaline lifestyle and avoiding items that have a high acidic content.

This diet plan requires you to consume alkaline producing food, while restricting or avoiding acid forming food. The proponents of this diet contend that an alkaline environment exists throughout your digestive tract, particularly within the intestine, which is where the majority of the digestive and absorption processes take place. Therefore, eating foods that are alkaline may help sustain that environment and promote the synthesis and activity of enzymes, both of which flourish in alkaline circumstances.

The primary tenet of the diet is based on a philosophical theory that asserts the foods we consume have the ability to readily affect the internal chemistry of our bodies. Everything hinges on whether the meal in question is acidic or alkaline. In a nutshell, the pH of our bodies will shift based on the meals that we consume.

Our bodies include organs that are efficient at getting rid of acid and neutralising its effects. There is a threshold beyond which our bodies are unable to adequately process any more acid. The alkaline diet does not aim to alter the pH level of the blood; rather, it relieves the strain of always striving to keep the body at a healthy pH level by providing it with the nutrients it needs to flourish. Foods that produce alkaline, such as plant proteins, tubers, vegetables, and entire fruits, are all alkaline due to the fact that they are anti-inflammatory, natural, fresh foods that are delectable and rich in antioxidants, chlorophyll, minerals, and vitamins. Other foods that form alkaline include whole fruits and vegetables. When a high concentration of alkalinity enters our circulation, it causes the formation of a barrier that works to maintain the health of our bodies. This barrier is called the alkaline buffer.

This is less of a diet and more of an eating plan than anything else. It is used in order to improve our health. After being absorbed and digested by the body, the food that we consume ultimately makes its way to the kidneys in the form of eight different chemicals that may either create a base or an acid. This diet places a strong focus on eating fresh fruits and vegetables.

There are a variety of methods that may be used to analyse meals and determine the amount of acid or base they provide to the body. Some foods are going to have a greater tendency to produce bases or acids than others. It may come as a surprise, but cheddar produces more acid than egg whites do. Spinach contributes more to the formation of bases than watermelon does.

Because of these factors, it is suggested that we make an effort to choose meals that have a high alkalinity content.

Consuming meals that are alkaline will neutralise the acid that is produced in the stomach, so making it simpler for the organ to digest food. Acid is produced not only by the stomach itself, but also by the digestion of a wide variety of acidic meals that must be taken and processed by the body. It is possible for the stomach to revert to its natural state of digestion and once again work at its peak capacity if acidic meals are avoided in favour of foods higher in alkaline content.

The alkaline diet is helpful in maintaining a consistent pH level in the body, which helps to prevent the hydrogen ions and proteins in the body from having their functions disrupted.

When a person eats, their bodies metabolise the food they take in and convert it into energy that can be used by the body. The purpose of the alkaline diet is to maintain the pH level of the body in a condition that is more alkaline, rather than acidic, and this is accomplished by encouraging the consumption of foods that are classified as alkaline. When trying to reach an alkaline state, the diet includes a detailed list of items that should be eaten and foods that should be avoided.

Because it encourages good biological functioning via the consumption of an appropriate food, adopting an alkaline diet is an essential first step towards leading a healthier lifestyle.

Why Is It So Difficult To Reduce One's Body Fat Percentage?

When energy is stored in fat, the volume required to hold it is reduced. If we were to store our energy in a different form, such as carbonhydrate, our overall mass would increase by a factor of two. One gramme of fat, for instance, has the capacity to retain 9 calories of energy, but one gramme of carbon hydrate or protein has only the capacity to store 4 calories. The main idea is that it is better to store energy in fat because it is more efficient.

Both acid and energy are stored in the body's fat stores.

Unfortunately, our fat stores are also the storage location for excess acid in our bodies. When the body is unable to completely eliminate the acid load, it will try to store any extra acid in a secure location. This is accomplished by the accumulation of fat. Acidic hydrogen ions are also stored in fat during the process of creating fat in order to act as a storage medium for energy. This contributes to the body's overall alkaline balance. If the acid load in the body is high when someone begins a diet in order to lose weight, it will be difficult to burn fat because the body will not want to release the acid that is stored in the fat depots. This makes it tough to burn fat. The body will fight against the process of burning fat. Burning fat, on the other hand, would not be as challenging for the same individual if they had alkali in their diet in order to reduce acidification. The presence of the alkali will be sufficient to neutralise the acid that is produced when fat is burned. When the atmosphere is alkaline, it is simpler to burn fat.

The trap of insulin resistance, shown in diagram form:

Oedema may be seen around the fatty tissues.

Water is stored in the areas of the body that have fat tissues. Around acidic tissues, there is a higher concentration of water, which helps protect against the harmful effects of acid. This condition is referred to as oedema. The high concentration of water exerts pressure on the region, which in turn causes the fat tissues to become compressed and restricts the passage of blood and lymph between them. When this occurs, there is a greater challenge in getting lipids to the liver. However, in order to be converted into usable energy, they first need to go to the liver and then the muscles. It is more difficult to burn fat when blood and lymph flow are reduced, as is the case when oedema is present.

When there is not enough alkalinity in the body, sugar is substituted for fat as the source of energy production.

The metabolism of a healthy individual who does not have an excessive amount of acid load can convert the fat, sugar, and protein included in meals into usable forms of energy. When there is a high acid load in the body, it is difficult for the metabolism to utilise fat for the creation of energy. Because getting energy from proteins leads to increased acidity in the body, sugar is the only other option left as a source of fuel for the body. Because of this, in an acidic body, sugar is used for the generation of energy rather than fat or protein. However, this results in an even greater rise in acidity and establishes a virtuous loop, increasing the likelihood that the body will produce energy by relying on sugar. The most significant contributor to acidity is found in the form of simple sugars.

A higher insulin level is the direct result of eating sugar. In spite of insulin's best efforts to bring blood sugar levels down, the body continues to rely on sugar as its primary source of fuel because it is unable to convert alternative fuel sources into usable energy in a timely manner. The amount of sugar in the blood lowers suddenly, resulting to an increased demand for sugar and an increased desire for sugary foods. By consuming foods high in alkalinity, we may put an end to these desires and reduce our consumption of sugar. Consuming foods high in alkalinity enables the body to make better use of fats as a source of energy.

The depletion of oxygen in tissues that results from acidification.

When tissues get acidified, the amount of oxygen they contain drops, while the amount of oxygen rises when alkaline foods are consumed. Without oxygen, the burning of fat is impossible. In the absence of oxygen, the cells will turn to sugar as their primary source of energy. The presence of oxygen in the blood and tissues is increased when an alkaline environment is present.

Maintaining an alkaline atmosphere is one of the most crucial aspects of effective breathing. Lactic acid is generated within the body whenever sugar is burned in the absence of oxygen. The tissues become more acidic as a result of lactic acid's presence.

During exercise, lactic acid is produced by the muscles. If you exercise at a high enough intensity for your muscles to use up all of their stored energy by using all of the oxygen that is available, then your muscles will start creating energy without oxygen. This results in the creation of lactic acid. The muscular spasms and aches that result from lactic acid are caused by the acid itself. During exercise, it is essential to maintain proper breathing since doing so enables the body to maintain an alkaline environment, which in turn helps to delay the creation of lactic acid.

The Differences Between Heartburn, Acid Reflux, And Gastroesophageal Reflux Disease

These three phrases are often used synonymously, yet they each have a very specific connotation in the English language. Acid reflux, also known as gastroesophageal reflux disease (GERD), is a chronic form of acid reflux that may range in severity from moderate to severe. Acid reflux is fairly prevalent. One of the signs and symptoms of each of these illnesses is heartburn.

Acid indigestion

This word is not accurate since the source of the discomfort associated with heartburn is not the heart; rather, it is the digestive system, and more particularly, it is centred in the oesophagus. The name "heartburn" is thus highly misleading. The most prominent symptom of heartburn is a burning sensation in the chest, which may range from moderate to severe in intensity and is often misdiagnosed as a heart attack.

Because the lining of the oesophagus is not as tough as the lining of the stomach, acid may induce a burning sensation in the oesophagus. Some individuals describe the pain as being acute, while others say it feels like it's burning, and yet others say it's like their chest is squeezing. It is possible for it to migrate up the oesophagus to the region of the throat or the neck, and it may feel as if it is just behind your breastplate at that point.

The majority of individuals get heartburn after eating and then lying down, and leaning over might make the discomfort more worse. It is estimated that approximately 60 million people in the United States experience symptoms of this illness at least once every month. Managing heartburn may be accomplished in a number of ways, including the following:

Giving up smoking

Dropping some pounds

Reduce your consumption of foods high in fat.

avoiding meals that are both acidic and hot.

Heartburn that is moderate and does not occur often may be treated with over-the-counter drugs such as antacids. However, if you find that you are using these medications several times per week, you should seek medical attention as this might be an indication of acid reflux disease or GERD.

Reflux d'acide

A circular muscle known as the lower esophageal sphincter (LES) connects your stomach to your oesophagus so that food and liquid may pass between the two organs. This muscle is supposed to tighten up the oesophagus after food has gone through into the stomach.

However, if it is weak or if it doesn't constrict as it should, stomach acid may travel back into the oesophagus; this condition is referred to as acid reflux.

Symptoms of acid reflux include:

Acid indigestion

The croup

A scratchy and painful throat

A flavour in your tongue that is either bitter or sour

A scalding sensation that is accompanied by a pressing sensation that moves down the breastbone.

What exactly is GERD?

Acid reflux disease, also known as gastroesophageal reflux disease (GERD), is a chronic form of the condition that occurs when someone has acid reflux two or more times per week or whose oesophagus becomes irritated. A diagnosis of GERD may be made when any of these conditions occurs. Leaving this untreated without seeking medical attention may result in long-term harm, which increases the risk of developing cancer.

Symptoms of GERD include:

Acid indigestion

Having bad breath

Teeth erosion as a result of an excessive amount of acid

Aching in the chest

A persistent hacking cough that won't clear up.

A sensation that the food or liquid that was previously in your stomach has moved up into your mouth or throat.

Symptoms of asthma

difficulties chewing and swallowing

Heartburn and acid reflux may both be caused by the foods that a person eats, as well as by lying down soon after eating. Many individuals experience both symptoms on a regular basis. On the other hand, gastroesophageal reflux disease, or GERD, is a persistent ailment that might be brought on by the following:

Overweight and obese

A hernia of the hiatus

Cigarette Use During Pregnancy

Drinking of alcoholic beverages

The lower esophageal sphincter (LES) muscle may be weakened by the use of certain drugs, including pain relievers, antidepressants, sedatives, calcium channel blockers, and antihistamines.

GERD has the potential to make your life difficult, but there are therapeutic options available, including the following:

Making adjustments to your diet

Dropping some pounds

Giving up smoking

Giving up drinking booze

There are several drugs that may lower the quantities of acid produced by the stomach.

The very worst option would be to have surgery to strengthen the LES muscle.

GERD is caused by a combination of a number of different conditions. These variables will lead to the LES being weaker, which will ultimately result in acid reflux becoming more severe:

The way of life, including smoking, consuming alcohol, being overweight, and having poor posture

Antihistamines, nitrates, theophylline, and calcium channel blockers are the medications that are used to treat this condition.

Diet - eating foods that are fried or high in fat, consuming coffee, tomatoes, foods with a mint flavouring, foods that are spicy, onions, garlic, and chocolate.

Behaviours regarding food consumption, such as overeating, eating too rapidly, and eating just before going to bed

a number of medical disorders, including diabetes, fast weight gain, pregnancy, and hiatal hernia

In the next few chapters, we will discuss some of the therapy alternatives, and then in subsequent chapters, we will discuss your nutrition.

The Never-Ending Cycle of Discord

how an overabundance of yeast might trigger cravings: An acidic way of life (and notably the usage of anti-toxins) will produce the underlying excess, which will therefore make supplement and energy deficiencies (B-nutrients, and so on), which will consequently lead a person to feel weak, depressed, and generally poorly. This results in a yearning, or in many instances an uncontrolled urge for items such as processed fat/sugar combination foods and stimulants to deliver a rapid "energy" (adrenaline) fix. These food sources that stimulate adrenaline production allow you to feel better quickly; nevertheless, the sugar stimulates the yeast, which causes it to produce more acid, which in turn further feeds the yeast, so making the problem worse. The cycle of unevenness continues, and the situation becomes worse with each rotation of the wheel. The most effective solution for this problem is to disrupt the cycle by adding more alkalinity and electrons to the environment. You can't resist the sugar need with willpower because it's mentally and emotionally taxing, and you can't kill the yeast since the yeast is your own cells in a muffled structure. You would prefer not to kill the yeast because the yeast is your own cells in a muffled structure.

You will essentially need to alter the surrounding environment in order to cause the yeast cells to die off or transform back into solid cells. Yeast is perfectly capable of thriving in an environment that is poor in energy and acidic. Therefore, all that is required of you is to reduce the amount of dead food you consume, get rid of the acid accumulation, and flood your body with electron-rich live foods. It is not enough to merely take supplements or treatments against communicable diseases; you must also modify the surroundings. Are you able to comprehend that recommending acidic antifungal medicine for athlete's foot or yeast infections is completely pointless?

The problem is in the line of thinking that leads us to conclude that these beings must be killed. Antibiotics are intended to fight illness, but they actually increase the likelihood of an overgrowth of yeast in the body. Antibiotics kill both beneficial and harmful bacteria (or, in reality, they don't kill anything; rather, they cause bacteria to transform in a way that makes them more dangerous, which can lead to secondary diseases), which is why, despite the fact that they may reduce the symptoms of an illness in the here and now, they can cause problems in the future. Homeostasis in the gut is necessary for the monitoring of yeast and other types of bacteria; however, if this equilibrium is disrupted, yeast and other types of bacteria can spread from the gut into the bloodstream. Shortly after finishing a course of antibiotics, individuals revert to the more traditional pattern of contracting germs such as colds, infections, coughs, and so on from other people and from the environment. Because of this, people have a tendency to grow immune to the effects of anti-biotics. When used in the appropriate context and after the underlying cause has been addressed, natural antifungals like some herbs may be extremely helpful in treating fungal infections. It is important to note that if a person has a yeast overgrowth, they will often and surprisingly be attracted to infectious foods like as mushrooms, yeast bread, and bear. This is something that should be taken into consideration. The yeast in the blood wants to make sure its travelling partners are comfortable, so it sends instructions to your brain to get you to consume particular foods so that its guests may complete their sacrifice. The list of illnesses that may be caused by yeast and other organisms is, in essence, never-ending. If you have a serious health problem, yeast might very well be a contributing factor in your condition. You can be absolutely assured of this. Many medical professionals are now aware of the relationship that exists between cancerous growths and yeast, as well as the fact that sickness is thought to be nothing more than a fungus or mould.

Let's face it, the most of us want to reduce our body fat first and foremost so that we may improve our appearance and then our overall health. When I first started, I was the complete opposite. I was already active and tried to maintain a diet that was relatively healthy, but as soon as I started college, I saw that I was having trouble maintaining my weight. My brother Carlo and I had agreed to improve our health and shed some pounds together, and judging by the letters he sent me, he was holding up his half of the agreement.

Unfortunately, it wasn't the case when I first started. However, things were different.

I committed myself fully to following The Alkaline Diet and did so as it was my work. Even the little shortcuts that were provided, such as drinking an alkaline-rich beverage before taking alcohol or caffeine, did not pique my curiosity. One example of this is drinking green tea. I just refrained from eating any of the items that were off limits. I even went back to the gym to do some weights. My first couple of occasions, I was under the impression that I would see Dwayne there. No, I did not. In point of fact, I did not run across him again. My best bet is that he moved schools or quit school altogether. I had the pleasure of meeting Stacey during one of my workouts. Stacey was the kind of girl whose body you'd give your life for if you had the chance. My whole life was turned upside down by just that one trip to the gym's weight room.

I discovered out that Stacey competed in the fitness industry, and wow, did she look the part! I found that I looked forward to working out more and more, but I never in my wildest dreams imagined that I would have a figure like

Stacey's. We began working out together almost immediately after we hit it off. Stacey ended up being the one who inspired me to keep going.

The Alkaline Diet that I was following was not nearly as complicated as Stacey's diet, which was. that was inevitable for that to be the case given that she was consistently training for a tournament. I followed my prescribed eating plan and exercise routine, and the results of both were visible in only two months' time. I wasn't the only one, and neither was anybody else. I did not go back to my hometown for the summer vacation between my sophomore and junior years of college. Instead, I decided to spend my time on college working on improving my physique. Not only had I shed a total of 70 pounds by the time I returned home for Christmas break during my junior year, but I had also significantly increased the amount of muscle that I had.

Carlo was my most successful opponent. As soon as he spotted me, he rushed over to me, wrapped his arms around me, and told me how proud he was of me. Even though he didn't look too bad himself, everyone in the neighbourhood was talking about how great I looked that year. Carlo did lose weight, but he wasn't as serious about it as I was, but I'm sure that when he saw me in person, a switch must have been flipped inside his brain that made him see how important it was to him. He was interested in learning more about the diet that I had followed to reach to this position.

I demonstrated everything to him. I demonstrated to him the foods that I consumed as well as those that I avoided. I told him that the reason I had decided to give The Alkaline Diet a try was because I had reached an extremely low moment in my life. I had to get moving straight immediately and accomplish something. I advised breaking it down into phases for Carlo, which contained the following items:

Being Aware Of What You're Consuming

We tend to cram food into our lips without giving much thought to the composition of the item we are consuming. Avoid eating items that contribute to the production of harmful acid in the body, such as refined carbohydrates, dairy products, meat, and fowl. These meals put a strain on the liver and kidneys, and they may even raise the chance of developing diabetes, which was already an underlying condition in our family. My doctor diagnosed me as having pre-diabetes many years ago. That was all it took for me to understand that this couldn't possibly be a joke any longer. I had no choice but to act immediately in response to it.

Knowing which foods contribute to an acidic environment and which ones contribute to an alkaline one is half the fight. It is possible that you may need to verify with a list at first, but after some time, it will become second nature. You'll find yourself in the supermarket, picking up the alkaline-promoting foods and drinks that you are certain will assist you in achieving your objective.

Apply the Rule of 2-to-1.

Follow this easy-to-remember guideline to get the most out of the meals that are high in alkaline minerals: for every item that is high in acid-promoting nutrients, consume two foods that are high in alkaline minerals. Here is a nice illustration:

Breakfast consists of acid-promoting eggs paired with alkaline-promoting vegetables, such as broccoli or spinach, and is accompanied with an alkaline-promoting half grapefruit. This method is effective, and you don't even have to give up eating the things you like the most—something I'm sure Carlo wouldn't do in any case.

Put Your Drinks Away Please

You may want to treat yourself to a glass of wine or soda once in a while with dinner, but try to limit how often you do so. That's not a problem. You may counteract the acid-producing effects of these foods by starting out with an alkaline beverage. To mitigate the side effects, try washing down some green tea with a lemon slice or a glass of water. (Keep in mind that you should use this in combination with the 2-to-1 Rule.)

Remember to Include Your Favourite Alkaline Spices and Herbs!

You may go ahead and treat yourself to some of those acid-promoting items now and again, but if you do, you might want to consider adding some alkaline-promoting spices for some flavour. You will achieve two goals at once by doing this; first, you will reduce the acid impact, and second, you will produce a meal that tastes fantastic. Do you like some soup or some nuts? Add some paprika to taste and sprinkle it on top. Mix one teaspoon of chilli powder into one cup of chocolate. (I gave it a go during the winter, and I really loved it!)

I briefed Carlo on all of these items and how the human body may be harmed as a result of consuming them in this manner. (Mom and dad even took a few notes throughout the lesson.)

My mother advised that I prepare the large Sunday meal that we always have, which consists of spaghetti and bread. It was necessary for me to take a few steps back since it seemed impossible that my mother would let anybody, and by that I mean anybody, into her kitchen. It was as if hell had to have frozen over first. After I had recovered from the first shock, I decided to make one of my go-to meals. This was my opportunity to persuade them to choose a different way of living. This must be of high quality.

This recipe was the closest thing I could come up with that reminded me of our old Italian dishes that were loaded with fat that we used to have for Sunday supper. What is the decision? It was a hit with them. Even after writing down the recipe, my mother vowed to prepare it for me whenever I returned home. (To this day, she has not changed her mind on it. (You're welcome, mum!)

APPROVAL BY THE GENERAL PUBLIC AND VERIFICATION OF THE FACTS

People who are interested in trying an alkaline diet should be aware that many medical professionals, nutritionists, and naturopaths consider these diets to be nothing more than a passing trend. It is significant that neither the National Centre for Complementary and Integrative Health (NCCIH) nor the Academy of Nutrition and Dietetics (AND) listed alkaline diets on their respective websites. Although the overall results of a diet high in fruits and vegetables and low in fats and refined sugar are beneficial for weight loss and heart health, responsible practitioners of naturopathy point out that the theory that underpins alkaline diets contradicts everything that is known about the chemistry of the human body. The U.S. News & World Report Health gave alkaline diets a poor grade (2.4 out of a possible 5) owing to the various arbitrary restrictions placed on food choice as well as the lack of data supporting the diet's claims.

As of the year 2018, there have only been a handful of mainstream clinical research conducted on alkaline diets, alkaline water, and other dietary supplements. As of the beginning of 2018, the National Institutes of Health have filed four separate research on alkaline water. In one piece of study, alkaline water was investigated as a potential sports beverage, while in another, it was investigated to see whether or not drinking alkaline water reduces skin toxicity in patients undergoing radiation therapy for breast cancer. In the other two studies, researchers investigated the effect that drinking alkaline water had on the pH level of human urine.

ALKALINE: KEY WORDS AND TERMS

The acid-ash hypothesis was an obsolete medical idea that incorrectly connected excessively acidic foods to osteoporosis and other harmful effects on one's health. The theory states that eating high-protein foods such as meat, poultry, fish, and other foods that burn to produce acidic ash causes the body to attempt to reduce the amount of acid by taking calcium from bone, which in turn causes the bone to become weaker and increases the chance of developing osteoporosis.

The maintenance of a constant pH level in the extracellular fluid (ECF) of the organism is referred to as acid-base homeostasis. The proportion of the human body's total water content that is found in extracellular fluid is about one-third.

Ash: Ash, as used in analytical chemistry, refers to the residue that is solid, non-gaseous, and does not contain any liquids after a substance has been entirely burnt. The evaluation and analysis of the material's metal and mineral composition is the goal of reducing the substance to ash.

A bomb calorimeter is a kind of equipment that maintains a constant volume and is used to determine the amount of heat produced by the combustion of a certain chemical. In the process of determining the amount of calories contained in food, bomb calorimeters are often used.

A plant belonging to the Fabaceae family is referred to as a legume. Among the legumes that are cultivated for grain seeds and fodder for cattle, some of the most common are chickpeas, alfalfa, lentils, clover, peas, beans, soybeans and peanuts.

Water, natural foods, herbs and other dietary adjustments, massage and manipulation, and electrotherapy are all examples of treatments that fall within the purview of naturopathy, an approach to illness treatment that prioritises the use of natural methods of health care above conventional medications and surgical procedures.

The pH scale is a quantitative scale that is used in the scientific discipline of chemistry. This scale is used to represent the acidity or alkalinity of an aqueous (water-based) solution. Acidic solutions have a pH value that is less than 7, whereas alkaline solutions have a pH value that is more than 7. The pH of pure water is 7, which indicates that it is in a neutral state.

Tofu is a kind of soft food that may be made by first coagulating soymilk with an enzyme, calcium sulphate, or organic acid, and then pressing the resulting curds into blocks or pieces. Tofu is often used in vegetarian and vegan cooking as a substitute for meat and dairy products.

www.ingramcontent.com/pod-product-compliance
Lightning Source LLC
Chambersburg PA
CBHW051732020426
42333CB00014B/1272